How I Eat Without Wheat

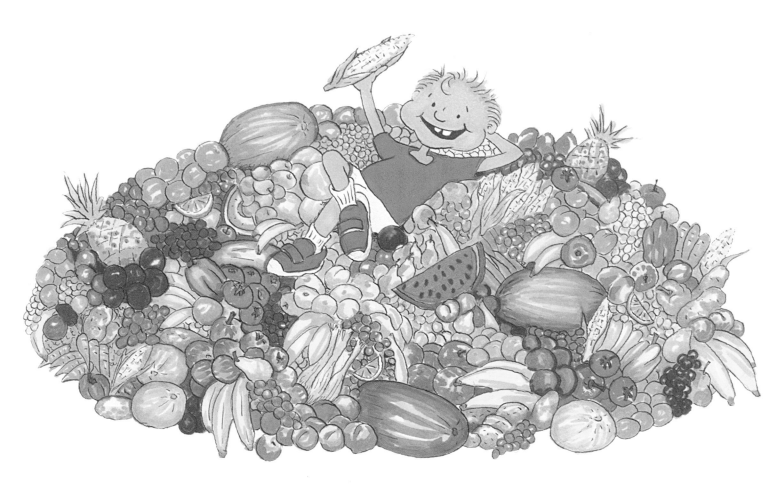

by
Karen Fine

Illustrated by
Russ Novak

AuthorHouse™
1663 Liberty Drive, Suite 200
Bloomington, IN 47403
www.authorhouse.com
Phone: 1-800-839-8640

AuthorHouse™ UK Ltd.
500 Avebury Boulevard
Central Milton Keynes, MK9 2BE
www.authorhouse.co.uk
Phone: 08001974150

First published by AuthorHouse 2/21/2007

ISBN: 978-1-4259-7570-8 (sc)

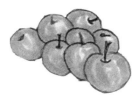

Library of Congress Control Number: 2006910897

Printed in the United States of America
Bloomington, Indiana

This book is printed on acid-free paper.

Bloomington, IN   Milton Keynes, UK

authorHOUSE®

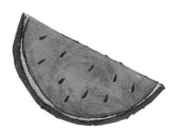

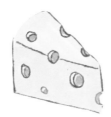

For Jack

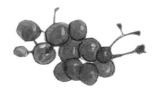

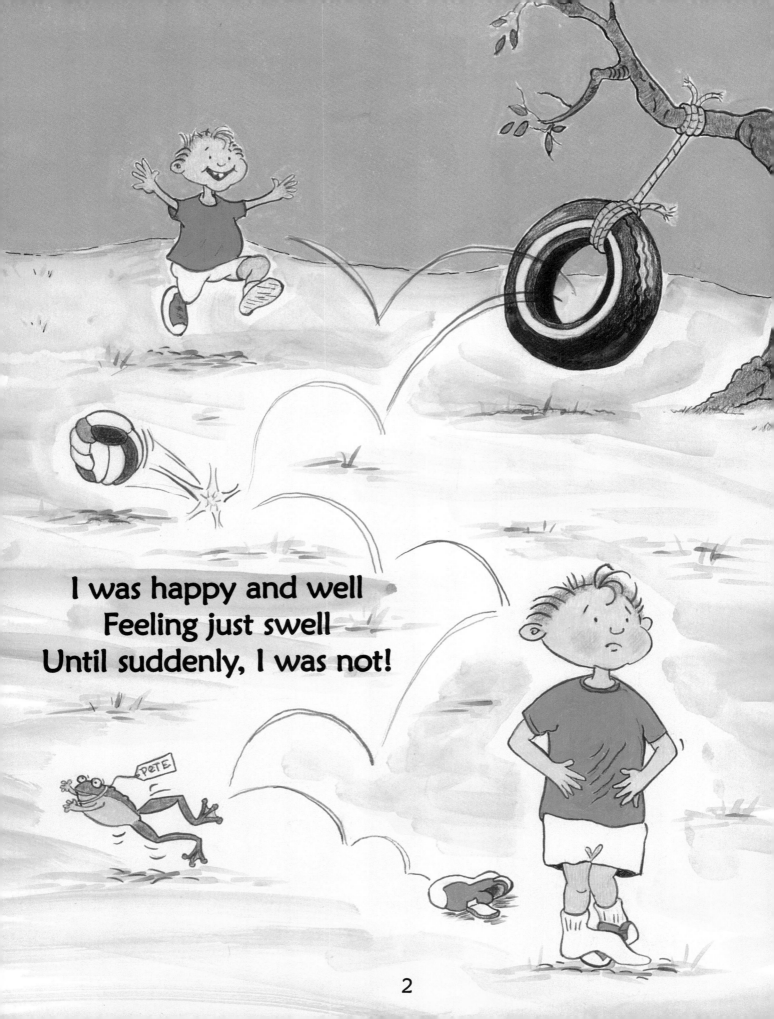

I was happy and well
Feeling just swell
Until suddenly, I was not!

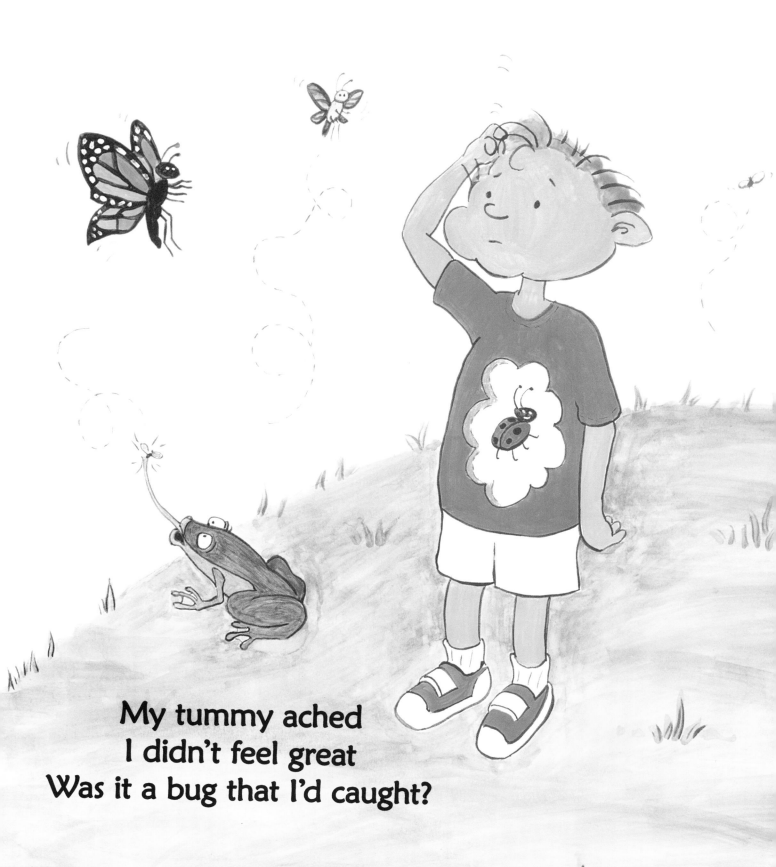

My tummy ached
I didn't feel great
Was it a bug that I'd caught?

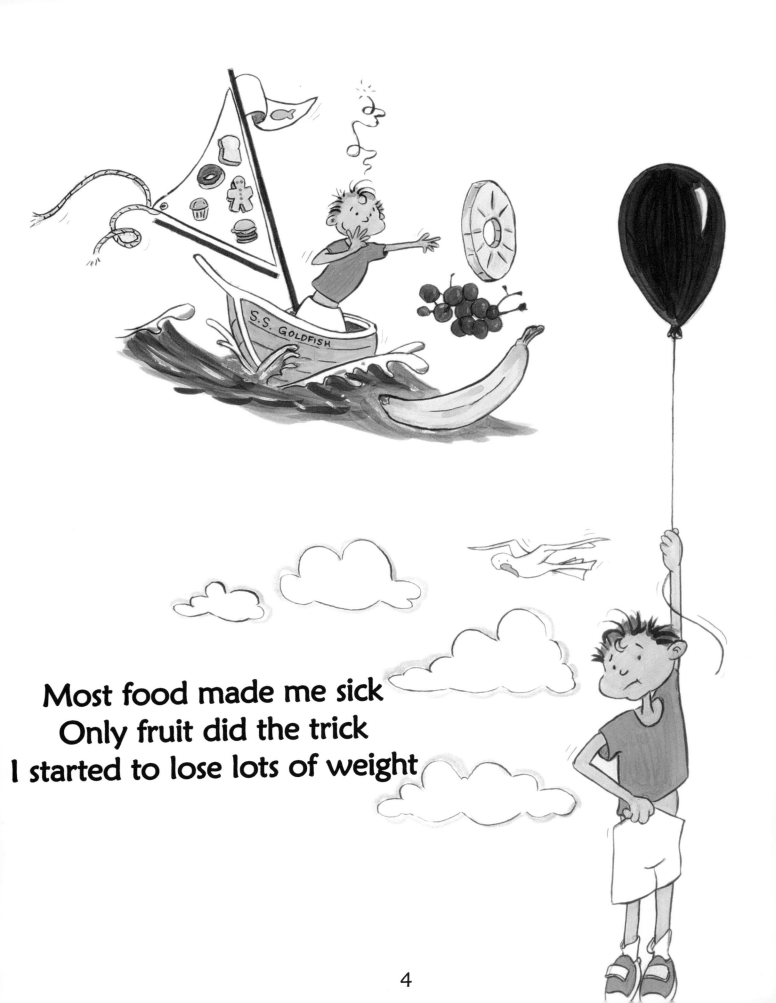

Most food made me sick
Only fruit did the trick
I started to lose lots of weight

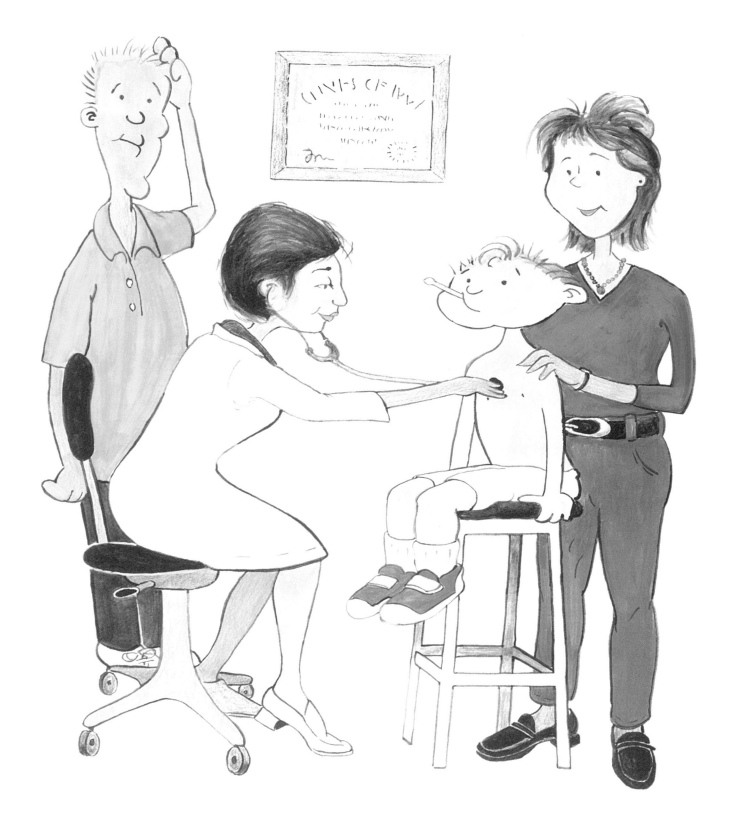

We went to the doctor
My parents had sought her
For help to learn my fate

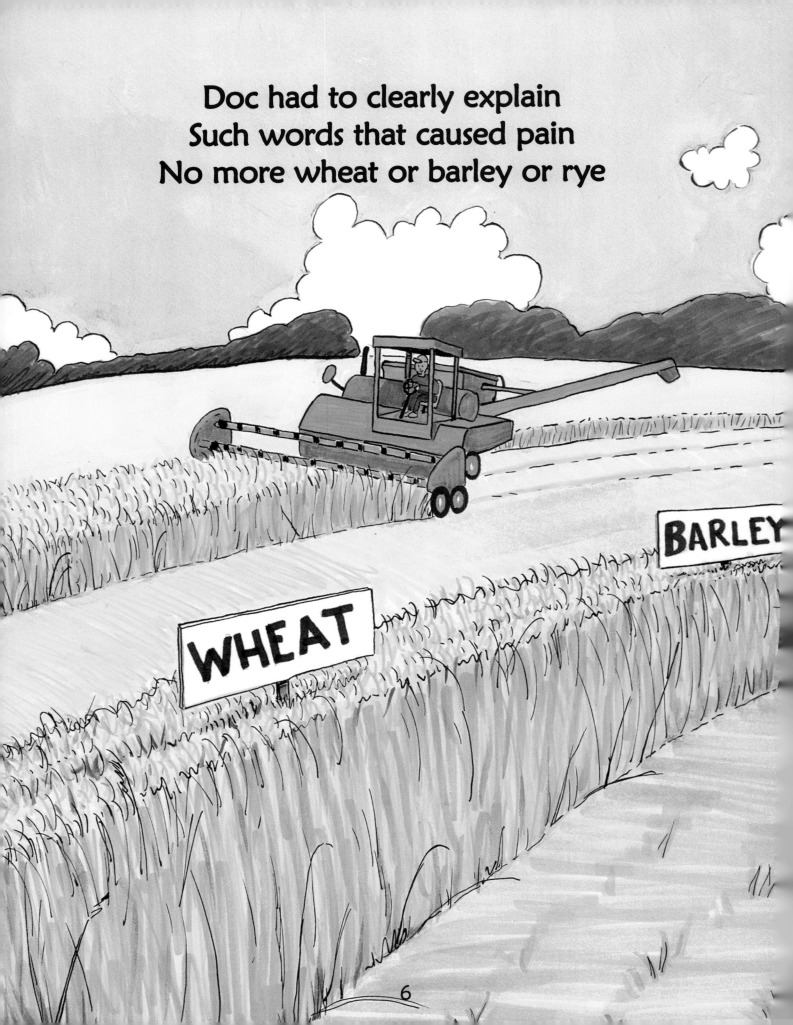

Doc had to clearly explain
Such words that caused pain
No more wheat or barley or rye

Until there's a cure
There's a way to be sure
No gluten, and I will see why

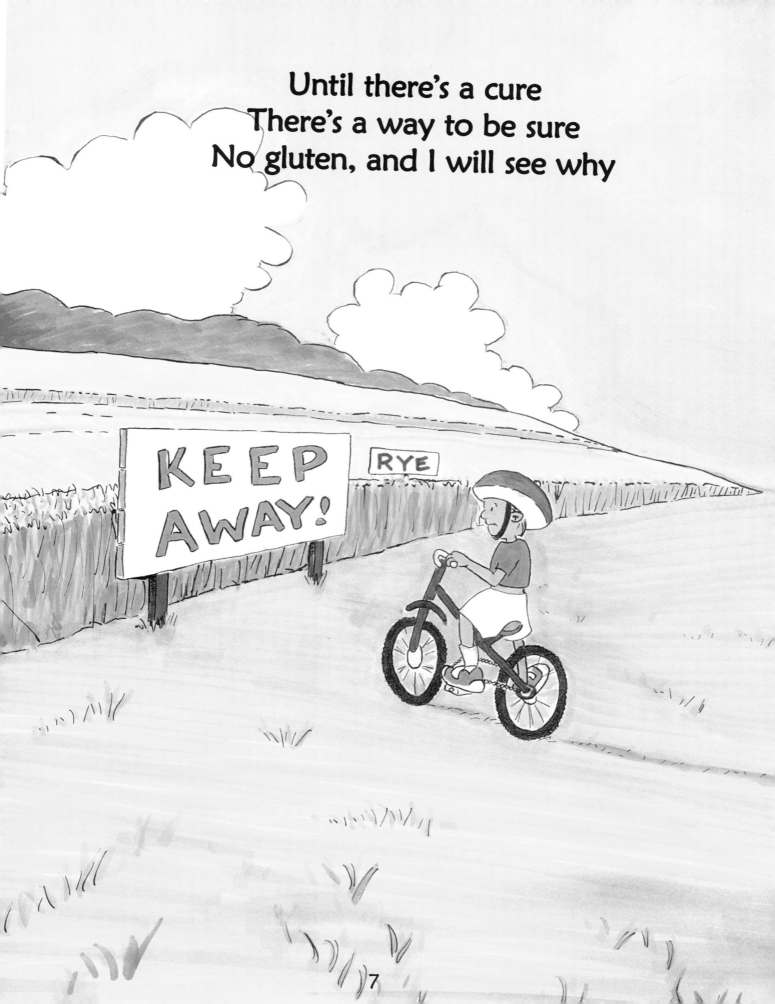

What's a parent to do?
They thought it all through
And went out and researched it all

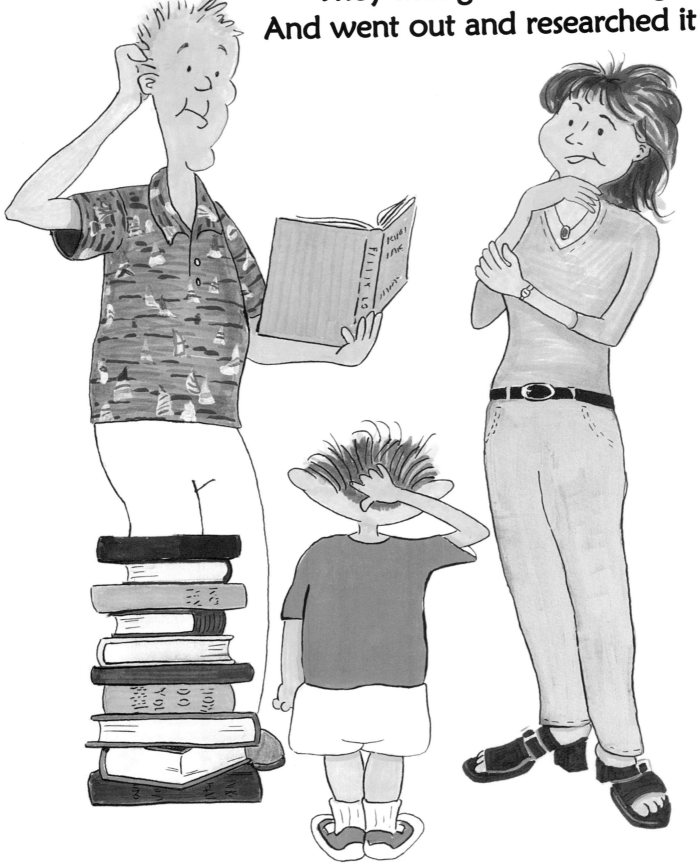

They searched high and low
And found places to go
To get food that would make me grow tall

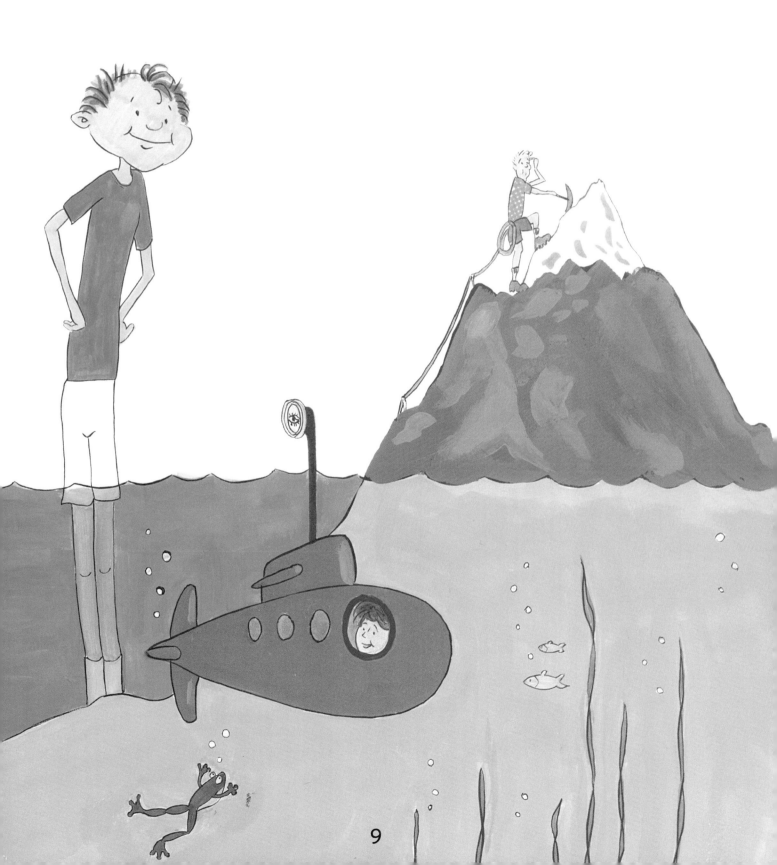

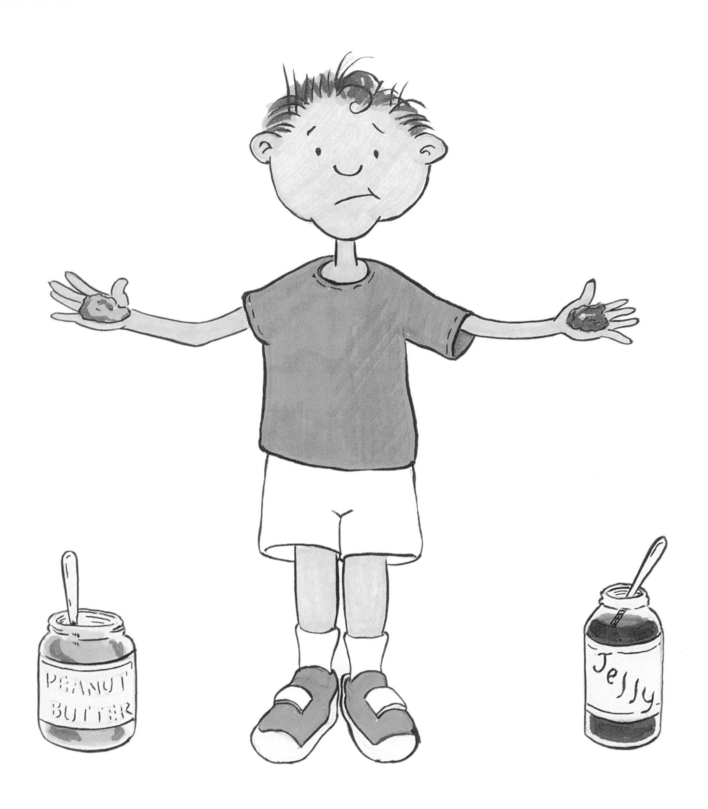

It was hard at first
No bread was the worst
But they found plenty of choices for me!

Bread, pasta and rolls
Doughnuts with holes
Made with special flour, you see

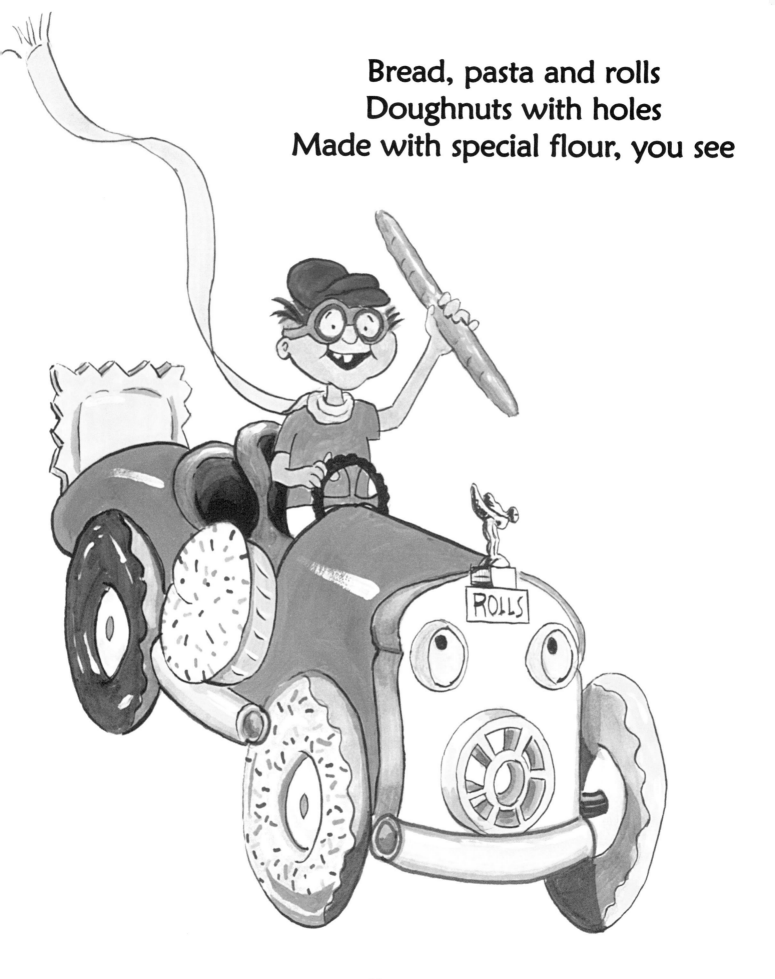

Meat, fruit and cheese
As much as you please
Spaghetti and sauce, why not?

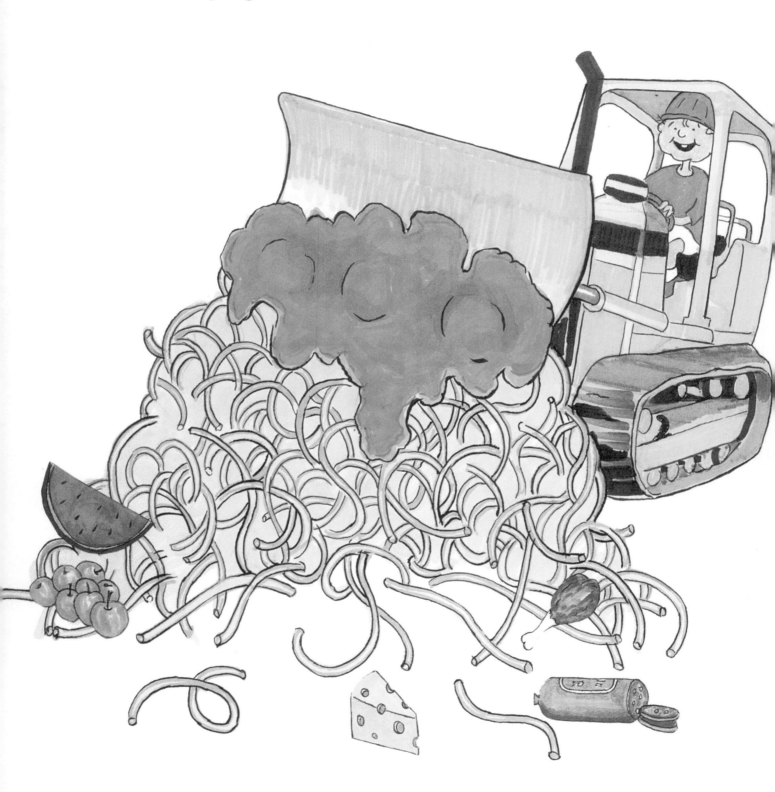

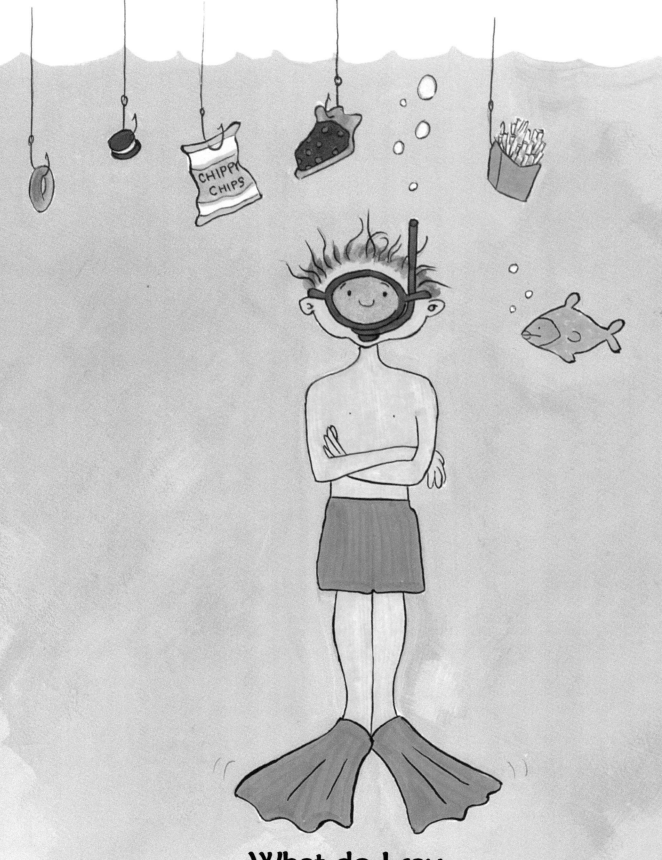

What do I say
When kids come my way
Offering me treats that they've got?

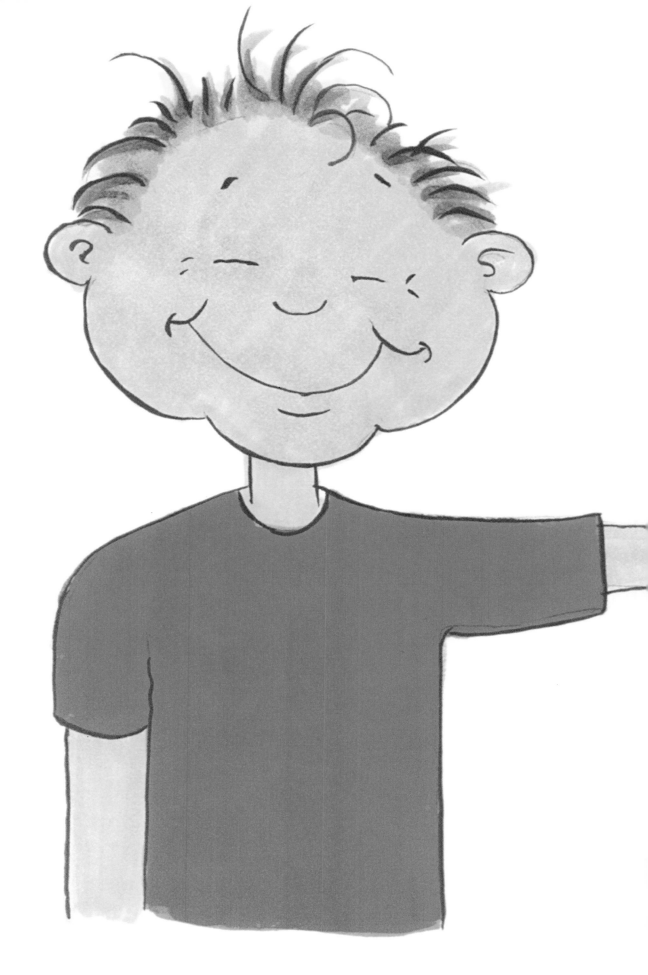

I give a big grin
Say, "No thank you" and then,
I am sure not to make a big deal

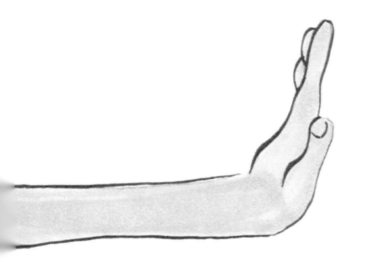
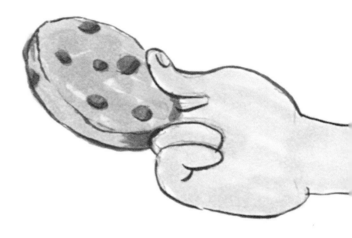

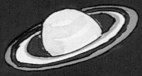
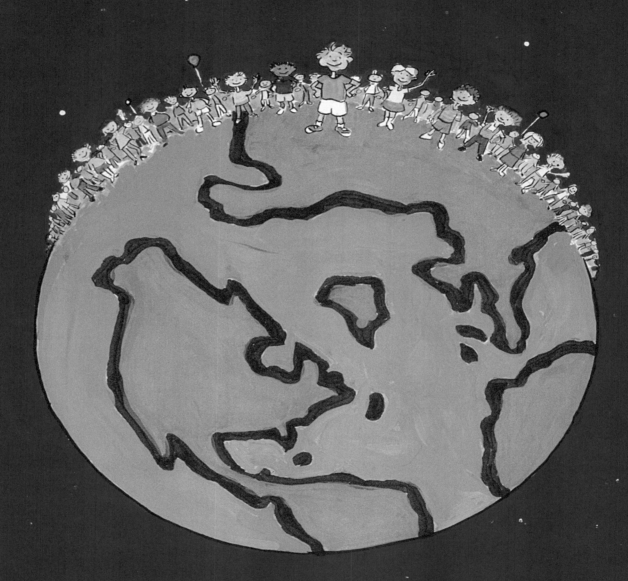
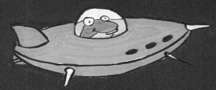

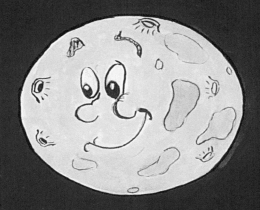

We've all got something you see
And there are more kids like me
Who can't eat some things with their meal

My new diet is great
I'm gaining weight

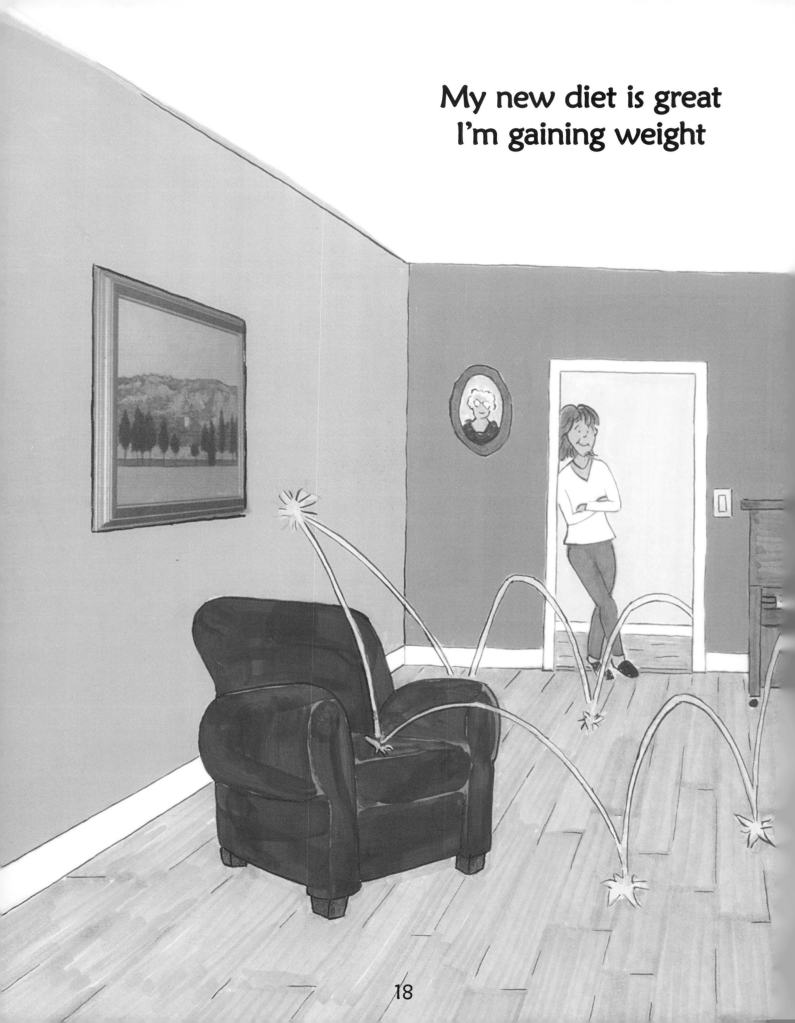

My mom says I
bounce off the walls!

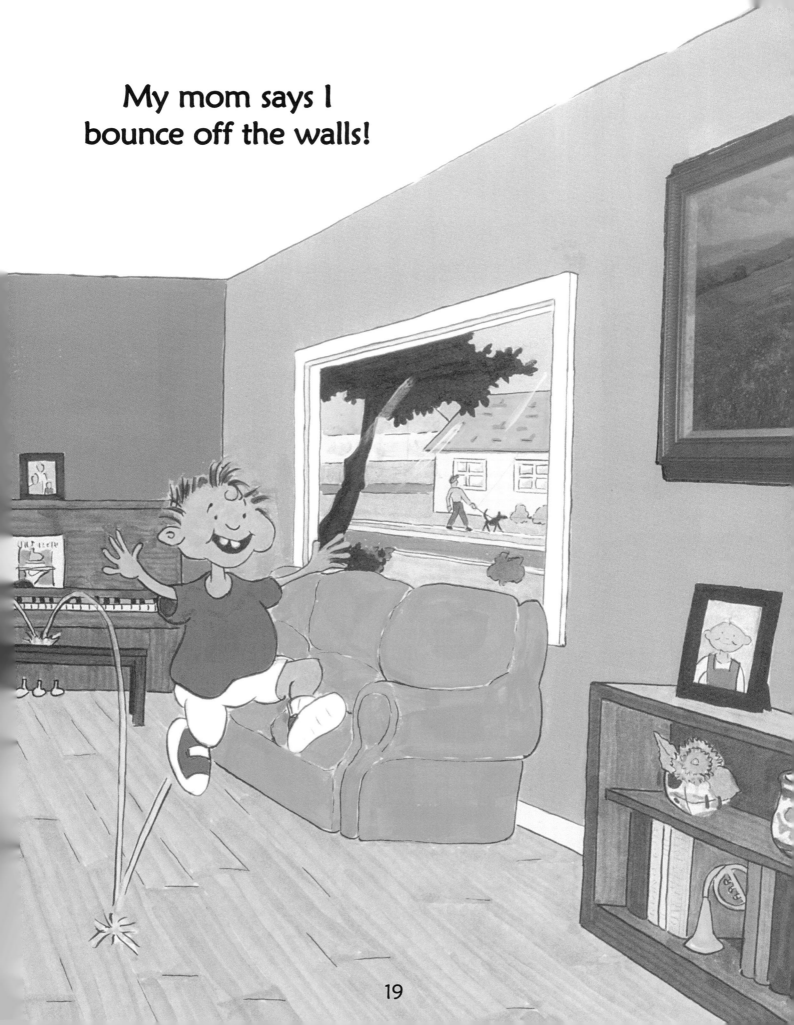

I'm feeling healthy and good
Like little kids should
My family is thankful and all

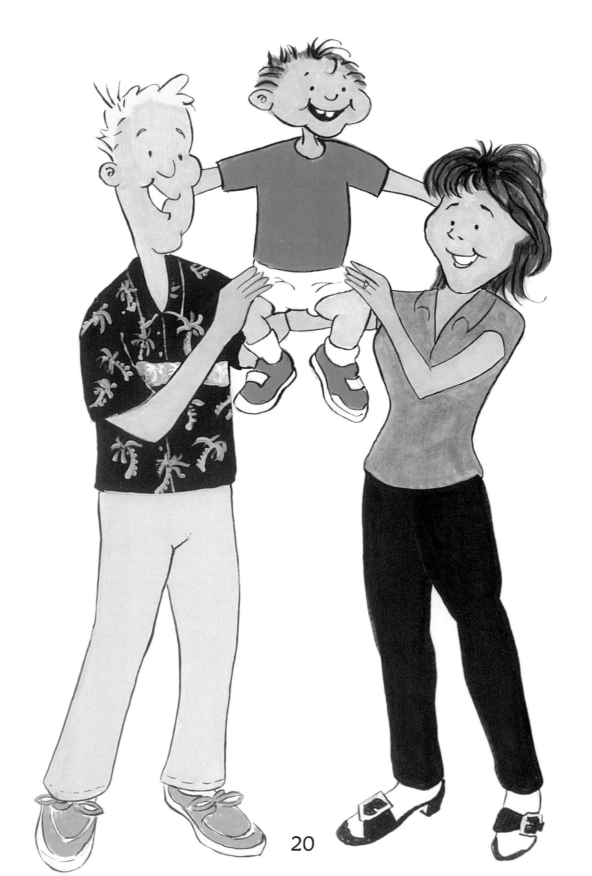

I have cake, it's true
And can now eat it too
My doc, I was lucky to meet!

I eat gluten free
It's so easy you see
And that's how I eat without wheat!

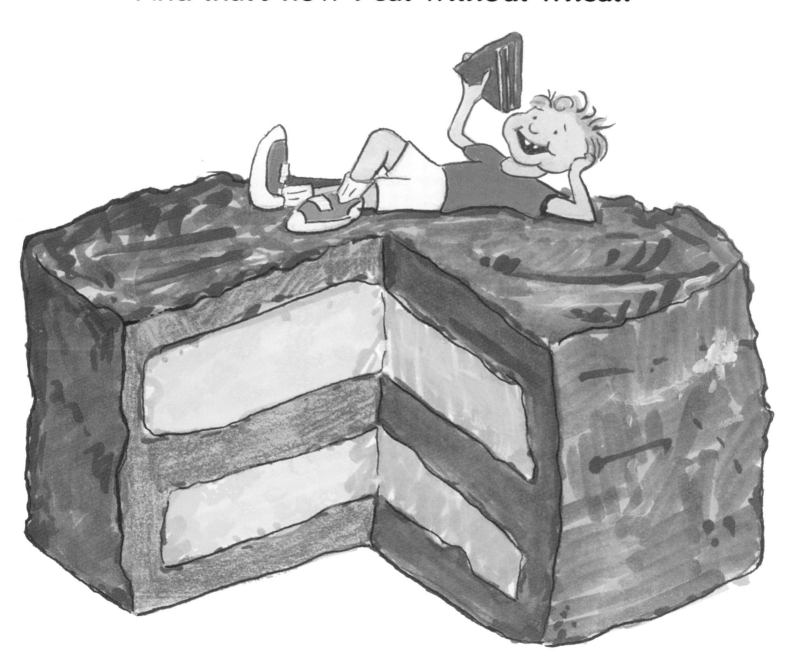

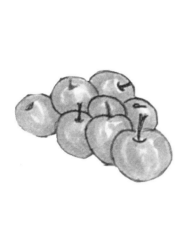
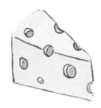
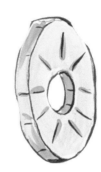

The End

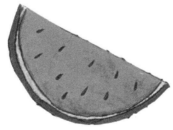
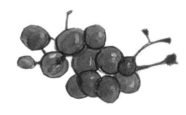